GLUTEN FREE

Carl Preston

© **2015 Carl Preston**
Edited by: Carl Preston
Cover by: Carl Preston

All rights reserved. No part of this publication may be reproduced, stored in a retrieval system, or transmitted in any form or by any means, electronic, mechanical, recording or otherwise, without the prior written permission of the author.

Whydontyouchange.com   2015

First Edition

Table of Contents

1 Gluten-free Zucchini Pies 2

2 Gluten-Free Banana Cinnamon Bread 3

3 Gluten-Free Chia Cookies 4

4 Gluten-Free Chocolate And Pumpkin Pies 5

5 Gluten-Free Almond Honey cake 6

6 Gluten-Free Buttery Peanut pie 7

7 Gluten-Free Sweet Corn Muffins Or Bread 8

8 Gluten-free Sugary pancakes 9

9 Gluten-Free Banana Cake 10

10 Gluten-free Coconut And Banana cakes 11

11 Gluten-free Berry With Pancakes 13

12 Gluten-free Pasta And Bacon Salad 14

13 Gluten-free And Low-fat Brownies 15

14 Gluten-free Beef And Tomato Pizza 16

15 Gluten-Free Pumpkin Chocolate Chips 17

16 Gluten-free Chocolate Banana Cakes 18

17 Gluten-Free Oats And Banana Muffins 19

18 Gluten-Free Banana Chocolate Cakes 20

19 Gluten-free Vanilla Granola Bars 21

20 Gluten-Free Fried Potato Pancakes 22

21 Gluten Banana And Oats Chips 23

22 Gluten-free Chocolate Brownies 24

23 Gluten-free Buttery Peanut Pies 25

24 Gluten-free Sautéed Shrimp 26

25 Gluten-Free Blueberry And Banana Muffins 27

26 Gluten-free Vodka Tortellini Sauce 28

27 Gluten-free Chocolate Egg And Walnut Cookies 29

28 Gluten-Free Baking Bread Powder 30

29 Gluten-Free Flour Mix for Muffins, Breads, Cookie Bars 31

30 Gluten-Free Flour Mix for Baking Cakes & Cookies 32

31 Gluten-Free Brown Bread Baking Flour Mix 33

32 Gluten-Free All-Purpose Baking Flour Mix 34

33 Gluten-Free Lemon-spiced Honey Chicken 35

34 Gluten-free Skillet potato cakes 36

35 Gluten-free Family Rice Cereal 37

36 Gluten-Free Cheesy Bread 38

37 Gluten-free Baked Taco 39

38 Gluten-free Banana Butter bread 40

39 Gluten-free Oven Fried Chicken And Cheese 41

40 Gluten-free Spicy Cheese Pizza 42

41 Gluten-free Fish Tacos 43

42 Gluten-free Bacon And Swiss Pie 44

43 Gluten-free Strawberry Coconut Milkshake 45

44 Easy Gluten-Free Butter Bread 46

45 Healthy Gluten-Free Chocolate Cookies 47

46 Gluten-free Shortbread Cookies 48

47 Gluten-free Wheat Corn And Apple Crumble 49

48 Gluten-free Dairy Coconut Cornbread 50

49 Gluten-free Pan-Fried Chicken 51

50 Gluten-Free Peanut Butter Oats 52

THE GLUTEN FREE DIET RECIPES

1 Gluten-free Zucchini Pies

Ingredients
- 4 Eggs, whisked
- 4 cups shredded zucchini
- ½ cup butter or ghee, dissolved
- 4 cups Almond flour
- 3 teaspoon Cinnamon
- ½ cup Honey
- 1 teaspoon Salt
- 1½ teaspoon Baking soda

Preparation
1. Get the shredded zucchini and dissolved butter ready and leave to stand.
2. Combine the almond flour, honey, dissolved butter, and zucchini together in a bowl.
3. Stir in the cinnamon, whisked eggs, soda and salt and mix properly.
4. Line the inside of the muffin tins with silicone or parchment paper and bake for approximately 20 minutes at 180°C.
5. Allow to cool then serve.

2 Gluten-Free Banana Cinnamon Bread

Ingredients

1st Batch
- 4 Mashed Bananas
- 1½ cup Canola Oil
- 8 Eggs

2nd Batch
- 3 cups Gluten Free Self Raising Flour
- 1½ cup Castor Sugar
- 3 teaspoon Bi-Carb
- 1 tablespoon Cinnamon
- ¾ cup Coconut

Preparation
1. Preheat the oven to about 160° degrees
2. Pour together the first batch of ingredients in a medium-sized mixing bowl and combine thoroughly.
3. Stir in the second batch of ingredients into the bowl of first batch, and pour in the flour last.
4. Transfer the mixture into two loaf tins lined with foil.
5. Bake for about an hour or until a toothpick inserted into the middle comes out clean.
6. Allow the loaves to cool completely before separating them from tins. Toast with butter and serve.

3 Gluten-Free Chia Cookies

Ingredients

Wet ingredients
- 100g Light brown sugar
- 150ml Water
- 2 tablespoons Chia seed
- 3 tablespoons Oil

Dry ingredients
- 50g Cocoa powder
- 70g Rice flour
- ½ teaspoon Baking powder
- 30g Ground Almond

Preparation
1. Saturate the Chia seeds in water.
2. Preheat the oven to about 180 °C. Evenly rub oil in the baking dish.
3. Combine the dry ingredients together in a bowl.
4. Combine the wet ingredients together in a blender or food processor until smooth. Now Pour the wet mixture into the bowl of dry mixture and stir together using a spoon.
5. Pour the mixture into a mini cup cake tin and bake them in the oven for about 20 minutes at 180°C until the surface hardens.
6. Once the exterior becomes a little hard, it's well done! Please consume within 2 days or refrigerate.

4 Gluten-Free Chocolate And Pumpkin Pies

Ingredients
- 1 cup White Chocolate Chips
- 3 cups Pamela's Baking and Pancake Mix
- 1 teaspoon Baking Powder
- ½ cup Sugar
- 1 cup Milk
- 1 teaspoon Cinnamon
- ¾ teaspoon Pure Pumpkin
- 1 teaspoon Nutmeg
- ¾ cup Pure Pumpkin

Preparation
1. Preheat the oven to 375 degrees. Combine together the dry ingredients in a bowl.
2. Stir in the milk and pumpkin, combining together properly to make the dough thick.
3. Mould large blobs of dough onto the evenly greased baking sheet and bake for about 17 to 20 minutes.

5 Gluten-Free Almond Honey cake

Ingredients
- 1½ teaspoon Baking soda
- 4 Eggs
- 1½ cup Glutinous Rice Flour
- 1½ cup Sugar
- 1 teaspoon Baking powder
- 1 cup Honey
- 1½ cup Coconut Flour
- 2 cups Oil
- 3 teaspoon Elite Instant Coffee Powder
- 1 teaspoon Cinnamon
- 1 teaspoon Xanthum Gum
- 2 cup Almond or Soy Milk

Preparation
1. Combine in a bowl, the honey, eggs, sugar and oil and until it becomes fluffy.
2. Stir in the almond or soy milk
3. Pour in the rest ingredients and stir together again.
4. Bake for about 45 minutes or until a toothpick inserted in the middle comes out clean.
5. You can sprinkle honey onto the cake to give it a honey flavor when serving.

6 Gluten-Free Buttery Peanut pie

Ingredients
- 2 Eggs
- 1½ cup Sugar
- 2 cup2 Peanut Butter

Preparation
1. Combine the ingredients in a bowl.
2. Heat it in the oven at 350 degrees for about 8 -10 minutes. Serve.

7 Gluten-Free Sweet Corn Muffins Or Bread

Ingredients
- 3 big eggs
- 2 cups gluten free flour
- 2 tablespoons sugar
- 1½ cup milk or almond or soy
- 2 tablespoons baking powder
- 1 cup corn meal
- 1 cup vegetable oil
- 1 teaspoon salt

Preparation
1. Mix together all the ingredients in a bowl and whisk together. Transfer into greased muffin tins or baking dish.
2. Bake for about 20 minutes in a muffin tin and 40 minutes in a baking dish at 350 degrees until the bread rises back up when slightly pressed in the center.

8 Gluten-free Sugary pancakes

Ingredients

Pancake batter
- 4oz water
- 1½ teaspoon baking powder
- 2 eggs
- 4oz rice flour
- 1 teaspoon sugar

Topping
- 1½ tablespoon honey
- Powdered sugar

Preparation
1. Combine all ingredients together in a mixing bowl. Heat the nonstick pan on medium heat add batter the mixture flipping the same way you do to a pancake.
2. Top with honey or powdered sugar or any other topping you desire.

9 Gluten-Free Banana Cake

Ingredients
- 4 bananas
- 190grams brown sugar
- 190grams self raising gluten-free flour
- 3 eggs
- 4 tablespoon vegetable oil
- 1 teaspoon bicarbonate of soda
- 80grams yoghurt
- 120grams chocolate or milk or dark

Preparation
1. Preheat the oven to about 180 degree Celsius. Line the inside of a 20 X 10 cm loaf tin with foil or parchment paper.
2. Mash the banana and combine with the brown sugar in a mixing bowl.
3. Stir in the eggs, flour, yoghurt, oil, and bicarbonate of soda. Mix together completely.
4. Shred or slice the chocolate and pour it into the mixture.
5. Transfer into the loaf tin and bake for about an hour until it turns golden and becomes springy.

10 Gluten-free Coconut And Banana cakes

Ingredients

Pancakes
- 4 tablespoon coconut flour
- 2 large ripe bananas
- 1 tablespoon grated dried coconut
- 3 large eggs
- Butter (for greasing)
- 1 teaspoon baking powder
- 1 tablespoon ground cinnamon

Topping
- ½ cup raspberries
- ½ cup blueberries
- ½ cup fresh cherries
- ½ cup water
- ½ cup honey
- ½ cup strawberries

Preparation
1. Add all the topping ingredients to a small pan and let it boil until the desired consistency. Reserve
2. Smash the ripe banana to get a banana paste.
3. In a separate bowl beat the eggs well.
4. Add the banana, the coconut flour dried coconut and ground cinnamon to the eggs.
5. At the end add the baking powder and mix well.
6. Heat and grease a skillet and bake about one scoop of the pancake mix at a time. This recipe should be good for about 6 pancakes.
7. When the pancakes are ready serve them with the berries topping

11 Gluten-free Berry With Pancakes

Ingredients
- 1½ teaspoon baking powder
- 2 cups gluten-free flour
- 2 tablespoon Agave syrup or honey
- 3 tablespoon Olive oil
- 1 teaspoon baking soda
- 3 eggs
- 1 teaspoon sea salt
- 1½ cup berries, optional

Preparation
1. Heat the saucepan on medium heat on a stove or heat griddle.
2. Combine the dry ingredients together in a bowl.
3. Whisk the eggs, and stir in the remaining wet ingredients into another bowl.
4. Mix together all the ingredients and pour in the berries. Mix them together.
5. Prepare the pancakes as usual. Serve with cinnamon, butter and sugar mixture.

12 Gluten-free Pasta And Bacon Salad

Ingredients
- 15oz package gluten-free rotini
- 2 cups matchstick carrots
- 10oz frozen peas
- 2oz Hormel Applewood smoked bacon
- ½ cup mayonnaise
- 1 cup Hidden Valley light Ranch dressing

Preparation
1. Boil the pasta by following the instructions on the pack.
2. Pour the frozen peas into a colander and drain the boiled pasta on top.
3. Place the peas and the pasta in a big mixing bowl and stir in the rest ingredients.
4. Refrigerate till ready to serving.

13 Gluten-free And Low-fat Brownies

Ingredients
- 3 egg whites
- 1¼ teaspoon vanilla extract
- 1 pack gluten-free brownie mix
- ½ cup fat-free plain yogurt

Preparation
1. Combine together all the ingredients and blend well. The batter will be solid. Spread the batter in 13x9x2 pan.
2. Bake in the oven for about half an hour at 350°F until it becomes solid.

14 Gluten-free Beef And Tomato Pizza

Ingredients
- 2lb ground beef
- 4 cups gluten-free baking mix
- 18oz Tomato sauce
- 2 cups water
- 1 teaspoon salt
- ½ cup butter
- 3 cloves garlic, grated
- 10oz grated Mozzarella cheese
- 1 teaspoon Italian seasoning

Preparation
1. Heat the oven to about 425 degrees. Evenly grease the casserole dish.
2. Combine the water, baking mix, and butter together until soft dough is formed. Place the dough in the bottom of the dish.
3. Heat and stir in the garlic, ground beef, and salt, until the beef turns brown, drain it out of the liquid and leave it to stand.
4. Combine the tomato sauce with the Italian seasoning and spread it uniformly on top of the dough. Drizzle the beef mixture uniformly over the sauce and garnish with cheese.
5. Bake for about 20 minutes until the crust becomes a golden brown color.

15 Gluten-Free Pumpkin Chocolate Chips

Ingredients
- 6 Eggs
- 1½ cans Pumpkin
- 1¼ cup Quick oats
- 1¼ cup Brown rice flour
- 1 tablespoon Baking powder
- ½ cup Honey
- 3 tablespoons Stevia
- 1 cup Chocolate chips
- ½ cup Almond milk
- 1 tablespoon Vanilla
- 2 tablespoons Cinnamon
- 1 tablespoon All spice

Preparation
1. Mix the ingredients together and then pour into the buttered cupcake pans for making muffins.
2. Bake for about half an hour at 350° degrees.
3. Turn off the heat, remove muffin from the oven and serve.

16 Gluten-free Chocolate Banana Cakes

Ingredients
- 1½ cups gluten free flour
- 2 eggs
- 3 teaspoons baking powder
- 3 tablespoons Gluten free flour
- 1 tablespoon Maple syrup
- 3 large ripe bananas
- 1 cup chocolate chips
- 2 teaspoon vanilla extract
- 1 teaspoon baking soda
- 1 dash salt

Preparation
1. Preheat the oven to 350°. Mash the bananas and egg together in a bowl. Stir in the maple syrup, vanilla, and salt and whisk together again until it is well blended.
2. Stir in the baking powder, flour, and baking soda. Mix together with the banana mixture and pour in the chocolate chips.
3. Rub grease in a 17 x 11 cookie sheet. Pour in the cake mixture and spread uniformly.
4. Bake for about 13 to 20 minutes. Slice into squares when it's cooled. Keep in sealed container in the refrigerator.

17 Gluten-Free Oats And Banana Muffins

Ingredients
- 4 Eggs
- 1¼ teaspoon Baking powder
- 1½ cups Quick oats
- 2 Bananas
- ½ cup Honey
- 1 teaspoon Vanilla
- 4 tablespoons Stevia
- 1¼ teaspoon Cinnamon

Preparation
1. Mix together all the ingredients in a blender or food processor and blend until it is well combined.
2. Switch the oven to 350 degrees and pour the blended batter into a muffin pan.
3. Put the muffin pan inside the oven and bake for about 20 to 30 minutes.
4. Remove when properly baked and serve.

18 Gluten-Free Banana Chocolate Cakes

Ingredients
- 3 Eggs
- 2 Bananas
- ½ cup Quick oats
- ½ cup Chocolate chips or unsweetened carob chips
- 1¼ teaspoon Honey

Preparation
1. Mix together all the ingredients aside from the chocolate chips in a blender or food processor and blend on high speed until it is smooth.
2. Then stir the chocolate chips into the batter and pour it into a pan and bake the pancakes over medium heat.
3. Toss after a few minutes or when one side of the pancakes becomes set.
4. Bake to desired doneness. Top with fruit if you prefer, and then serve!

19 Gluten-free Vanilla Granola Bars

Ingredients
- 1 cup coconut oil
- ½ cup pure maple syrup
- 2 cups gluten-free rice krispies cereal
- ½ cup brown sugar
- 3 cups gluten-free quick oats
- ½ cup chia or hemp or flax seeds
- 1½ teaspoon vanilla extract
- 1½ cup dried cranberries
- Mini chocolate chips
- Pinch sea salt

Preparation
1. Line foil inside an 8x8 baking pan and grease evenly.
2. Combine honey, coconut oil, vanilla extract, and brown sugar in a pot.
3. When properly mixed, switch the heat to medium-high and allow the mixture to boil for a minute.
4. Turn off the heat and stir in the rest ingredients, aside from the chocolate chips.
5. Press the mixture tightly into the pan, stir in the chocolate chips, and press again.
6. Refrigerate for about 2 hours, then take it out and slice to any size you prefer.
7. Keep in a sealed container for about one week.

20 Gluten-Free Fried Potato Pancakes

Ingredients
- 2 cups leftover white potatoes, mashed
- 1 big egg
- Ghee or butter, for frying
- ½ cup Gluten-Free All-Purpose Flour
- ¼ cup scallions, diced
- Sour cream and chives for serving, optional
- Pepper and salt to taste

Preparation
1. Mix together all the ingredients in a big mixing bowl. Combine properly.
2. Dissolve the ghee or butter in a skillet over low-medium heat.
3. Divide the pancakes using an ice cream scoop or a half-cup dry measuring cup.
4. Spoon the divided mashed potatoes into the pan, 2 at once, and use a spatula to squash to preferred thickness.
5. Cook each side for about 5-6 minutes or until it turns golden-brown and flop over.
6. Turn off the heat and serve at once with chives and sour cream, if preferred.

21 Gluten Banana And Oats Chips

Ingredients
- 2½ cups Gluten-free oats
- 4 Bananas
- ½ cup Soy milk
- 1¼ teaspoon Ground cinnamon
- ¾ teaspoon Vanilla extract
- ½ cup Applesauce
- ¾ cup Dairy-free chocolate chips

Preparation
1. Pre-heat the oven about to 350° Fahrenheit
2. Squash the bananas completely until it becomes smooth.
3. Pour the wet ingredients into the squashed bananas first.
4. Stir in the dry ingredients next.
5. Toss the mixture until the chocolate chips and oats are uniformly coated.
6. Scoop the batter onto the cooking sheet using a spoon or ice cream scoop and spread it out at two inches from each another.
7. Bake for about 20 to 30 minutes.
8. Allow the cookies 10 minutes to harden a bit.
9. Store the cookies in a sealed container and refrigerate till ready to consume.

22 Gluten-free Chocolate Brownies

Ingredients
- 3 eggs
- ½ cup soy flour
- 1 teaspoon baking soda
- ½ cup cornstarch
- ¾ cup butter
- ½ cup unsweetened cocoa powder
- 1¼ cup packed brown sugar
- ¾ teaspoon vanilla
- 1 cup semisweet chocolate chips
- ½ teaspoon salt

Preparation
1. Preheat the oven to abut 350°F.
2. Spray nonstick cooking spray on 8" square baking pan.
3. Mix together the baking soda, flour, salt and cornstarch in a medium mixing bowl and combine thoroughly.
4. Dissolve the butter in a big skillet over low heat. Stir in the brown sugar; heat and whisk until the sugar melts. Turn off the heat; stir in the cocoa until it s well blended. Add the flour mixture and stir until smooth. Add the vanilla and chocolate chips. Pour in the eggs; whisk it until it becomes smooth and well mixed. Transfer into chosen saucepan.
5. Bake for about half an hour or until a toothpick inserted into the middle comes out almost clean.

23 Gluten-free Buttery Peanut Pies

Ingredients
- 3 eggs
- 2 dash ground cinnamon
- 3 cups granulated sugar
- 3 cups Creamy Peanut butter
- 1¼ teaspoon vanilla extract
- 1 tablespoon Salt
- 1 dash ground nutmeg

Preparation
1. Preheat the oven to about 350°F. Combine the vanilla, peanut butter, egg and sugar, in a small mixing bowl until well blended.
2. Scoop 1 tablespoon of the mixture which is roughly 1 inch separated onto the ungreased baking sheets. Press down the mounds using the tines of a fork, creating a crosshatch design on the cookies. Garnish the cookies with salt.
3. Bake the cookies for about 20minutes until it turns golden around the edges, changing the position of the sheets midway through baking. Remove and place on racks to cool.

24 Gluten-free Sautéed Shrimp

Ingredients
- 1lb medium to large-sized shrimp
- 2 eggs
- 1 cup oil for frying
- 3 teaspoon cayenne pepper
- 2 cups corn starch

Preparation
1. Rinse and devein the shrimp.
2. Heat the oil in sauce pan or wok over medium heat.
3. Crack the eggs into a bowl and whisk.
4. Toss the shrimp in the egg.
5. Combine cayenne and corn starch together.
6. Mix the coated shrimp with the corn starch mixture. Coat fully.
7. Stir-fry the shrimp until it turns golden brown on either side. Use tongs to carefully flip the shrimps.
8. Enjoy

25 Gluten-Free Blueberry And Banana Muffins

Ingredients
- 3 big Eggs
- 2¼ cups Gluten Free Flour
- 2 big Bananas
- 3 teaspoons Baking Powder
- ¾ cup melted Butter
- ½ teaspoon nutmeg, ground
- 1¼ teaspoon Vanilla
- 1 cup Sugar
- 3 cups Blueberries
- 1 cup Organic Milk
- 1/3 teaspoon Salt

Preparation
1. Combine the dry ingredients together in a bowl.
2. Combine the wet ingredients together in a bowl.
3. Don't add the Blueberries until you are almost done.
4. Using a mixer combine the wet and dry ingredients together and then add the banana.
5. When the mixture is smooth pour it into the Blueberries.
6. Pour into 18 separate cups or muffin tins
7. Bake for at least 40 minutes at 350°F.
8. Leave it to cool then serve.

26 Gluten-free Vodka Tortellini Sauce

Ingredients
- ½ box barillas penne gluten-free pasta
- 1lb shredded turkey
- 1 can classico vodka sauce
- 1½ cup spinach
- 1 pack gluten-free cheese tortellini
- 1 pinch Lawry's seasoned salt

Preparation
1. Shred the turkey.
2. Season it with Lawry's seasoned salt.
3. Boil the penne pasta and tortellini.
4. Pour in the vodka sauce to the shredded turkey.
5. Stir the spinach into the vodka sauce and shredded turkey mixture.
6. Drain the pasta from the liquid
7. Combine all the mixtures together and stir. Serve.

27 Gluten-free Chocolate Egg And Walnut Cookies

Ingredients
- 4 tablespoon warm water
- 2 tablespoons ground flax seed
- 3 cups almond flour
- 1 teaspoon baking powder
- 1 cup Nutiva extra virgin coconut oil melted
- ¾ cup creamy almond butter
- 2 teaspoons ground cinnamon
- 1 cup walnuts chopped up fine
- 2 teaspoon vanilla extract
- 1 cup semi sweet chocolate chips
- ¾ cup pure maple syrup
- ¾ teaspoon sea salt

Preparation
1. Mix together the water with the ground flax leave to stand.
2. Combine the remaining ingredients together and pour in the flax mixture.
3. Replace cover and refrigerate for about 2 hours or more.
4. Preheat the oven to 350 degrees.
5. To prepare the cookies, take spoonfuls of dough and roll into 1-inch balls and gently press with your hand and put it on the cookie sheet.
6. Bake the cookies for about 20 minutes until it turns lightly brown.
7. Leave it to cool fully before taking it from the cookie sheet.
8. Enjoy

28 Gluten-Free Baking Bread Powder

Ingredients
- 75grams baking soda or bicarb of soda
- 150grams white rice flour
- 75grams tartaric acid

Preparation
1. Combine the ingredients together and sieve multiple times.
2. Keep in a sealed jar.

29 Gluten-Free Flour Mix for Muffins, Breads, Cookie Bars

Ingredients
- 120grams cornstarch or potato starch (not flour)
- 150grams sorghum, brown rice flour or GF oat
- 50grams almond flour or quinoa
- 80grams cornmeal or buckwheat flour
- 80grams millet flour

Preparation
1. The GF flour is a bit heavier and more ideal for making cookie bars, breads and breakfast muffins.
2. Mix together the ingredients.
3. Divide into 5 or more cups and store in a sealed container.
4. Add half teaspoon of xanthan gum into every third of the mixture to prepare normal loaves, muffins or cookies.

30 Gluten-Free Flour Mix for Baking Cakes & Cookies

Ingredients
- 190 grams potato starch
- 150 grams sorghum flour
- 80 grams buckwheat or millet flour

Preparation
1. This mixture can be used in making breads but is more ideal for making cookies, muffins, cakes and cupcakes.
2. Simply mix together the ingredients.
3. Add 1 teaspoon of xanthan gum to 3 cups of flour.
4. Bake and serve. It can also be stored in the fridge for about 3 months.

31 Gluten-Free Brown Bread Baking Flour Mix

Ingredients
- 50 grams sorghum flour
- 100 grams rice bran or ground flax seed
- 400 grams potato starch
- 300 grams brown rice flour
- 120 grams tapioca starch or corn starch

Preparation
1. Mix together the ingredients and store in a sealed container.
2. It can be mixed together and baked into bread, muffins or cakes.
3. Serve and enjoy.

32 Gluten-Free All-Purpose Baking Flour Mix

Ingredients
- ¾ part brown rice flour
- 1 part corn starch
- ¾ part white rice flour
- ½ part millet flour
- 1½ part sweet rice flour
- 1 part sorghum flour
- 1 part potato starch

Preparation
1. Mix together all the ingredients until well combined and store in a sealed container in the refrigerator.
2. Shake properly before using and for each cup you use, stir in 1 teaspoon of potato flour and add xanthan gum.
3. You can use this recipe to replace any recipe for all purpose flour.
4. Use the recipe within a month of mixing before it loses its nutritional values.

33 Gluten-Free Lemon-spiced Honey Chicken

Ingredients
- 3lb Diced Chicken Breasts, shredded
- 1 tablespoon coconut oil
- ½ cup Lemon juice
- ½ cup coconut aminos
- ½ cup honey
- 3 tablespoons grated garlic

Preparation
1. Heat the coconut oil in a saucepan and stir-fry the shredded chicken until it no longer looks pink.
2. Combine the remaining ingredients together in a bowl.
3. Once the chicken is done, pour in the sauce mixture and boil for an extra 5 to 10 minutes.
4. Serve with rice and cooked broccoli.

34 Gluten-free Skillet potato cakes

Ingredients
- 5 big potatoes, chopped
- 1½ cup Bob's red hill potato flour
- 3 tablespoons parsley
- 4 tablespoons vegetable oil
- 2 small onions
- 2 cloves garlic

Preparation
1. Mix together all the ingredients aside from the potato flour in a food processor or blender and blend properly.
2. Transfer the mixture into a bowl of flour. You may add a little more flour till it is as thick as preferred.
3. Place the skillet over the stove and add the vegetable oil.
4. Use an ice cream scoop or spoon to transfer the mixture into the skillet.
5. Press down the mixture using a spatula to make a flat potato cake.
6. Toss the cake as you fry until it becomes golden Brown on both sides.
7. Serve and add salt to taste

35 Gluten-free Family Rice Cereal

Ingredients
- 2 eggs
- 3oz rice flour
- 1 quart oil
- 3oz water
- Sugar to sprinkle after frying
- 2 graters with small holes, not the box grater

Preparation
1. Combine the ingredients together for making rice crisp cereal, should be similar to pancake batter.
2. Heat the oil over 375 degrees of heat. Scoop the batter onto a flat grater over the hot oil, fry just before the color begins to change. Ensure the oil doesn't splash! Use a wooden slotted spoon or metal strainer to remove the crisp and place on a paper towel.
3. Sprinkle a little sugar on the Rice crisp and allow it to cool. Store in the fridge or consume like normal cereal!

36 Gluten-Free Cheesy Bread

Ingredients
- 3 Eggs
- 4 tablespoons Olive oil
- 200ml Milk
- 200grams Rice flour
- 140grams Potato flour
- 150ml Water
- 60grams cheese, grated
- 1 pinch Salt and pepper

Preparation
1. Warm up the milk, oil and water until it simmers.
2. Pour the flour in a bowl and pour in the boiled liquid. Then knead.
3. Pour in the eggs little by little and knead in between pours. Stir in the cheese, salt, and pepper.
4. Bake in an oven for about half an hour at 250°F.
5. Enjoy! Serve when it's still warm.

37 Gluten-free Baked Taco

Ingredients
- 1½ lb ground beef
- 2 cups gluten-free baking mix
- 20oz refried beans
- 1 cup Yellow cornmeal
- ¾ cup butter, dissolved
- 1 cup cold water
- 1 cup water
- 2 cups cheddar cheese, grated
- 1 sachet gluten-free Taco seasoning

Preparation
1. Heat the oven to about 425°F. Rub grease in the casserole dish.
2. Combine the cornmeal, baking mix, 1 cup of water, and the butter together. Spread at the bottom of the dish to form a layer. Bake for about 10 minutes.
3. Boil and stir the beef until it becomes brown; drain from the liquid. Add the taco seasoning and 1 cup of water. Heat to boiling point, stirring repeatedly. Lower the heat. Uncover and allow it to simmer for about 10 minutes, stirring repeatedly until it becomes thick.
4. Spread the beans over the baked crust. Drizzle with the beef mixture and top with the cheese. Bake for about 10 more minutes.
5. Garnish with your preferred toppings, such as taco sauce, tomato, lettuce, onions, sour cream, and so on.

38 Gluten-free Banana Butter bread

Ingredients
- 4 tablespoons peanut butter
- 4 tablespoons stevia
- 1½ cup instant oats
- 3 bananas
- 1 teaspoon powdered cinnamon
- 3 tablespoons favorite jelly
- 1¼ teaspoon baking powder
- 1 teaspoon vanilla extract

Preparation
1. Put all the ingredients together in a blender and blend until smooth (though the oats will make it a little bumpy).
2. Transfer the blended mixture into a microwave safe baking pan or cupcake mold and microwave for about 4 to 6 minutes. Enjoy!

39 Gluten-free Oven Fried Chicken And Cheese

Ingredients
- 8 chicken breasts
- 2 teaspoon paprika
- 1 cup gluten-free baking mix
- 1½ tablespoons butter, dissolved
- 1½ teaspoon salt

Preparation
1. Preheat the oven to 425°F. Pour the dissolved butter into the bottom of the baking dish.
2. Combine the paprika, baking mixes, and salt together. Toss the chicken in the baking mix mixture before placing it in the baking dish.
3. Bake for about 20 minutes before flipping it over and bake it for another 15 minutes. Allow it to set for 5 minutes. Serve.

40 Gluten-free Spicy Cheese Pizza

Ingredients
- 5 frankfurters, finely chopped
- 3 cups gluten-free baking mix
- 10oz chili
- 1 cup butter, dissolved
- 1 cup water
- 2 cups cheddar cheese, grated

Preparation
1. Preheat the oven to about 425°F. Rub the nonstick cooking spray on a cookie sheet or pizza pan.
2. Combine the baking mix, dissolved butter and water until it forms soft dough. Pour in a little extra water if required. Spread the dough into a 12-inch circle on the saucepan. Pinch the edge of the circle to form a rim.
3. Spread the chili over the dough. Garnish with frankfurters and top with cheese.
4. Bake for about half an hour until the crust turns golden brown.

41 Gluten-free Fish Tacos

Ingredients
- 4 tablespoon olive oil for frying
- 4 white fish filets
- 4 tablespoons water
- 2 tablespoons rice wine vinegar
- 2 cups cornstarch
- 4 limes
- 4 tablespoons olive oil
- 1 tablespoon onion powder
- 1 tablespoon cayenne pepper
- 1 tablespoon garlic powder
- 2 teaspoons coarse sea salt

Preparation
1. Combine the juice from the rice wine vinegar, limes, garlic, Olive oil, salt, water, cayenne, and onion powder together.
2. Heat the oil on medium heat.
3. Toss the fish filets in the corn starch generously.
4. Put the fish filets in the hot oil, and stir-fry for about 3 to 5 minutes until it becomes brown on both sides.
5. Stir in the wet mix to the filets and allow it to simmer for about 3 minutes on low heat.
6. Serve with Pico de gallo, white corn tortillas and shredded cheddar.

42 Gluten-free Bacon And Swiss Pie

Ingredients
- 8 slices bacon, boiled and shredded
- 1/3 cup gluten-free baking mix
- 1/4 teaspoon onion powder
- 3 eggs
- 1 cup soymilk
- ½ cup Swiss cheese, grated
- 1/8 teaspoon pepper
- 1/8 teaspoon salt

Preparation
1. Heat the oven to about 350°F. Rub grease on the pie plate.
2. Scatter the shredded bacon and cheese in the bottom of the pie plate. Mix the rest of the ingredients together for a minute before pouring it into the pie plate.
3. Bake for about an hour until it turns a golden brown color. Allow to cool for about 5 minutes, and then serve.

43 Gluten-free Strawberry Coconut Milkshake

Ingredients
- 500ml full-fat coconut milk
- 2 pink or red food dyes, if preferred
- 8 tablespoons strawberry nesquik milkshake powder
- 3 tablespoons cornstarch or corn flour

Preparation
1. Combine the cornstarch with a little milk to make slurry.
2. Heat the remaining milk with the Nesquik in a medium saucepan.
3. Once it's about to boil, stir in the corn flour slurry and continue stirring until it becomes thick. Boil for about 2 minutes. Include a drop of food dye to give it a brighter colour.
4. Allow to cool to room temperature before serving.

44 Easy Gluten-Free Butter Bread

Ingredients
- 2 tablespoon butter
- 1 cup gluten-free flour
- 1½ cup water
- ¼ teaspoon sea salt

Preparation
1. To prepare the flatbread combine in a bowl 1 cup of gluten free flour, ¼ teaspoon of salt and 1½ cup of water. Dissolve 2 tablespoons of butter over medium heat.
2. Pour the flour mixture into the pan and then promptly spread to cover the bottom.
3. Heat until the edges turn brown and then toss onto the other side. While frying you may need to turn over several times to brown uniformly.
4. To prepare this recipe vegetarian or dairy-free simply replace the butter with 1 tablespoon of olive oil.

45 Healthy Gluten-Free Chocolate Cookies

Ingredients
- 1 cup natural peanut butter
- 2 can chick peas, unseasoned. Washed and drained
- ½ cup honey, unfiltered, organic honey
- 2 teaspoons baking soda
- 3 teaspoons vanilla extract
- 1 cup Dark chocolate chips
- Coconut oil, for baking sheet

Preparation
1. Preheat the oven to 350 degrees.
2. Put all the ingredients, aside from the chocolate chips, in a blender or food processor and blend until it becomes smooth.
3. Stir in the chocolate chips.
4. Use a spoon to scoop mixture onto a uniformly greased cookie sheet.
5. Bake for about 15 minutes or until it turns brown.
6. Serve!

46 Gluten-free Shortbread Cookies

Ingredients
- 2 cups flour
- 2 cups butter, melted
- ½ cup cornstarch
- 1 cup confectioner's sugar

Preparation
1. Preheat the oven to 350 degrees.
2. Beat the butter to a fluff and then add other ingredients and stir together.
3. Heat on low heat for 1 minute, and then on high heat for another 3 to 4 minutes.
4. Bake for about 10 minutes and ensure the edges don't get overly brown.

47 Gluten-free Wheat Corn And Apple Crumble

Ingredients
- 150grams granulated sugar
- 150grams rice flour
- 3 big cooking apples
- 100grams margarine (dairy-free, Vitalite)

Preparation
1. Preheat the oven to about 190°c.
2. Skin, core and dice the apples and arrange in a cooking dish, drizzle with a little sugar.
3. Pour the flour and margarine into a mixing bowl and combine until it looks like breadcrumbs.
4. Pour the sugar into the bowl and mix ingredients thoroughly.
5. Spread the crushed mix on top of the apples.
6. Bake for about half an hour until it turns golden brown.
7. Serve with soy custard.

48 Gluten-free Dairy Coconut Cornbread

Ingredients
- 100grams sugar (optional, though it makes the cornbread smooth)
- 1½ cups cornmeal
- 100ml vegetable oil
- 1 cup rice flour
- 280ml light coconut milk or any milk of choice
- 1 cup cornstarch or corn flour
- 1 teaspoon xanthan gum
- 2 tablespoon baking powder
- 3 tablespoons ground chia or flax seeds combined with 8 tablespoons hot water or 3 eggs
- 1 teaspoon salt

Preparation
1. Allow the chia seed and water mixture to stand until it becomes gelatinous while you put on the oven.
2. Preheat the oven to about 400°F and rub grease on an 8-inch square cake tin or baking dish. Put the tin inside the oven and leave it to heat while you prepare the batter.
3. Next combine the dry ingredients in a medium-sized mixing bowl and stir in the oil, milk and chia mixture or 3 eggs until the batter becomes smooth. Set aside for 10 minutes.
4. Take out the hot tin from the oven and transfer the batter into it. Replace the tin in the oven and bake for about half an hour or until it turns golden brown on top.
5. Slice into squares, drizzle with maple syrup or honey if preferred and serve hot from the oven either.

49 Gluten-free Pan-Fried Chicken

Ingredients
- 150grams rice flour
- 2 big chicken breasts
- 2 tablespoon oil
- 2 eggs

Preparation
1. Shred the chicken into the preferred sizes and pour into a large mixing bowl.
2. Whisk the eggs and drizzle it over the chicken making sure it is well coated.
3. Pour the rice flour to the bowl and make sure the chicken is uniformly covered.
4. Pour oil into the saucepan, allow it to heat and then fry the chicken until it turns golden brown flipping repeatedly to make sure it is properly cooked.
5. Serve as preferred.

50 Gluten-Free Peanut Butter Oats

Ingredients
- 1¼ cups gluten-free rolled oats
- 2 big Bananas
- 1½ cups unsweetened almond milk
- ½ cup Creamy Peanut Butter
- 2 tablespoons chia seeds (optional)
- 1 teaspoon ground cinnamon
- 1 teaspoon vanilla extract

Optional Toppings
- 1 Dark chocolate shavings or chips
- 2 Bananas, chopped
- 1 Coconut shavings

Preparation
1. Mash the banana in a medium-sized bowl using a spoon or fork.
2. Pour the rest of the ingredients into the bowl and combine well.
3. Transfer the mixture into two sealed containers and store in a refrigerator for about 3 hours or overnight.
4. When prepared to serve, stir the oats properly, garnish with any toppings you desire!

Made in the USA
Middletown, DE
15 December 2016